The Magnesium Deficiency Crisis

IS THIS THE WORLDS NUMBER ONE MINERAL DEFICIENCY?

Peter Ochsenham & Professor Juergen Vormann

Peter Ochsenham & Professor Juergen Vormann

Published by madhouseMEDIA

Kindle Edition

Contents

*To every pregnant woman, every person who is at a
higher risk of heart disease, to every person susceptible to
type 2 diabetes and all who live under stressful conditions
or are near to burn out - let this book serve as a reminder
that diet is important and that magnesium is crucial for
your health and may even save your life*

Whatever the Father of disease is, ill diet is the Mother.

—Chinese Proverb

Foreword

Magnesium deficiency has the potential to affect each and every person even before they are born. Many of us have known for a long time that most of our modern diseases from cardiovascular issues such as heart disease, stroke, and congestive heart failure, to diabetes, cancer, osteoporosis, and autoimmune diseases the likes of Crohn's or rheumatoid arthritis are intimately linked to the industrial world's flawed eating habits. If whole populations again began to eat wild berries, roots, and nuts, together with free-ranging meats and wild seafood, much of the pharmaceutical industry and the medical field those aspects that deal with degenerative diseases would quite simply go out of business.

In this book we will elucidate with good science – why you need to be concerned with your magnesium levels, why there is widespread deficiency and what are the diseases associated to this deficiency and also the life threatening consequences of this deficiency.

This book will also provide an outline as to the different types of deficiency and even a questionnaire so that you may be able to see if you might need some magnesium in your diet.

Also in the resource section we will find links to video questions and answers on magnesium and magnesium deficiency.

We hope that this book serves as a reminder of the importance of our collective attention to diet. magnesium is an interesting topic because its deficiency is so widespread and the consequences are so vast and as said many times during the book have a life and death consequence.

We cannot understand why for instance magnesium is not the frontline treatment for migraine or why anyone with signs of heart disease are not instructed immediately to supplement their diet with either magnesium rich foods or a magnesium supplement. We wonder how many lives could be saved.

We hope you enjoy the book – and it serves as a wonderful reminder of the immense power you have over your own health

The Crisis of Magnesium Deficiency

The importance of magnesium for our bodies is so crucial that it's surprising how neglected this amazing mineral was during the last century of research. Some scientists even refer to magnesium as the "forgotten ion." During recent years, however, many new aspects of magnesium have been discovered, and it was discovered that this essential mineral in particular has a tremendous impact on our disease risks, as well as our life expectancy.

Magnesium is found widely in nature. Indeed, it's the eighth most common element in the earth's crust. So it's not surprising we also find a high concentration of this element in the oceans—55 mmol per liter. (In the Dead Sea in Israel, the concentration of magnesium is extremely high, nearly 200 mmol per liter.) Since life evolved in seawater, quite simply, magnesium has been present throughout our evolution, with the result that no cell on earth can live without it. In virtually no physiological process is this mineral unneeded.

The human body contains around 25 grams of magnesium, distributed in such a way that a little more than half is found in our bones—53% to be precise. The bones act as a storage facility for magnesium.

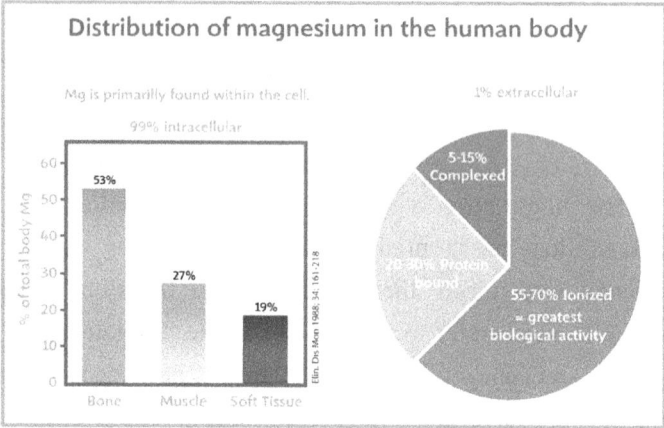

Figure 1: distribution of magnesium

[3]

What are the main physiological functions of magnesium?

One of the most important functions of magnesium is in it's complex with ATP (adenosine triphosphate), which is our intracellular fuel. This fuel is active in the form of the ATP-magnesium complex. If we take magnesium away, we can't use our ATP any longer, which means that an intracellular magnesium deficiency leads to an energy deficit in the cells. Magnesium is also crucial to the mitochondria, which are a membrane-enclosed structure found in cells. The mitochondria function as "cellular power plants," generating ATP.

Although allowing us to use intracellular fuel is a fundamental function of magnesium, it's far from the only function of this vital mineral. For instance, magnesium is also physiological antagonist to calcium and functions as a cofactor in more than 300 enzymes. As such, it's essential to various structural proteins, as well as the structure of nucleic acids. Many important enzymes require the proper concentration of intracellular free magnesium, and the body utilizes a variety of regulatory protocols to maintain the optimum concentration in our cells. But magnesium's extracellular function is also important.

In recent years magnesium has emerged as extremely important for the functioning of insulin, which means there's a close connection between magnesium and diabetes.

Further, it's known that magnesium has anti-apoptotic properties, which influence the processes involved in cancer. Probably as a result of its function in cell adhesion, magnesium deficiency plays an evident role in the spread of the cancer cells.

How Magnesium Does Its Work

How does magnesium work? There are several different mechanisms.

A cell membrane has a great many negative charges. As a divalent cation (an atom missing two electrons compared with a neutral atom), magnesium has two positive charges. By acting as a ligand—that is, a means of binding to two negative charges—magnesium stabilizes the cell membrane. This it does by cross-linking these charges.

If we eliminate magnesium or have a low extracellular concentration—in other words, a low concentration of magnesium in the plasma, the blood—these charges will bind sodium or potassium instead of magnesium. Both sodium and potassium are monovalent ions that cannot cross-link the membrane. Thus if we take magnesium out of the picture, we destabilize the cell membrane. This has especially important repercussions for the nervous system.

In a cell, magnesium is able to enter a calcium channel—although it's too big to pass through the channel. The result is that a certain percentage of the body's calcium channels are blocked by magnesium. The block isn't permanent but, as we shall see, serves a purpose for a time. The availability of calcium channels is determined by the quantity of magnesium present in the plasma.

This is a particularly important function of magnesium, given that calcium is used as a second messenger. Calcium channels are intimately linked with sodium channels in the cell membrane, which send a signal to the cell to release the stress hormones adrenaline and noradrenaline. The rapidity of this response, and the payload delivered, is greatly influenced by the amount of magnesium present. If a person has a magnesium deficiency, the calcium channel will transfer its signal more rapidly, thus releasing an excess of stress hormones—and doing so far more rapidly than were magnesium sufficiently present in the channel to partially block it and thereby regulate the rate of release. In other words, a high magnesium concentration slows the process, which means that magnesium is a natural anti-stress mineral—a truly important function and of particular significance for individuals in a stressed state.

A sufficient magnesium intake is crucial for the regulation of it´s homeostasis. Daily dietary intake of magnesium should be at least 300 milligrams, preferably more toward 420 milligrams, with 360 as a mean. Generally, only about a third of the magnesium we take in is absorbed in our intestines, with two-thirds remaining in the intestines—which is why an excess of some forms of magnesium in particular can cause diarrhea. After absorption, the blood distributes magnesium to the other cells; and if there is an increase, then the other cells can also fulfill their magnesium needs.

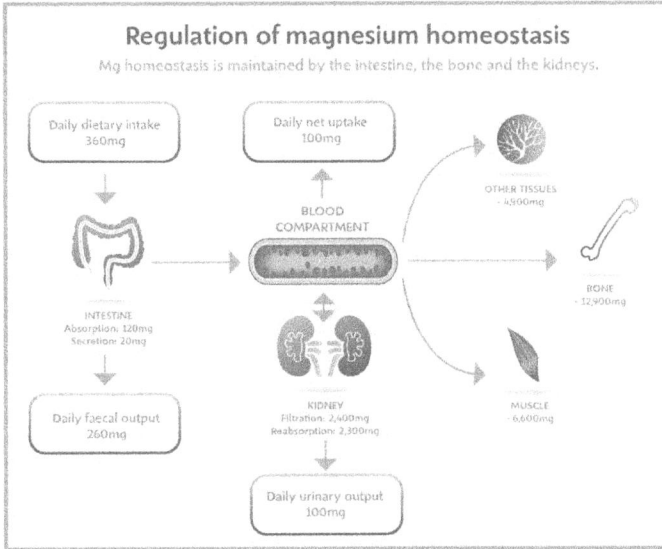

Figure 2: Regulation of magnesium homeostasis

The kidneys are the main organs in terms of regulating the homeostasis of magnesium in our bodies. Some 2,400 milligrams of magnesium are ultra-filtrated out of the blood by the kidneys on a daily basis, 95% of which must be reabsorbed from the primary urine. An adequate dietary intake provides us with a net uptake of around 100 milligrams from the intestines, one third of the daily dietary intake. To be in a steady state, or what we refer to as "homeostasis," we must excrete just these 100

9

milligrams, which we do through the urine. This means the individual has to reabsorb 2,300 milligrams of the 2,400 milligrams that enter the kidneys with the ultra-filtrate from blood. Hence the kidneys fulfill a vital role in regulating the amount of magnesium in the body. Everything that influences kidney function also influences the homeostasis of magnesium.

5

How Magnesium Is Absorbed by the Body

During recent years, the mechanisms by which magnesium is absorbed in the intestines and reabsorbed in the kidneys have become clear. Having said this, we need to point out that when it comes to science, it's always more complicated than the simple statement that something is "clear." With this proviso in mind, several mechanisms are nevertheless known to us.

We have two different pathways for the absorption of magnesium. The first is via para-cellular pathways, which are a pathway that crosses a layer **between** cells, and for this we need the so-called Claudins—proteins that decide whether magnesium can pass into the blood. These proteins are under the control of vitamin D. Thus a vitamin D deficiency affects the homeostasis of magnesium. Even if you receive a lot of sun, a deficiency of vitamin D isn't at all uncommon.

Another pathway is trans-cellular, meaning transport **through** the cells. There are several cellular channels for magnesium uptake. Although these are the most important channels, other transporters also bring magnesium into the cell. However, we don't require magnesium only in the cells; we need it in the blood, and beyond. For this we need a different system. This is the so-called sodium-magnesium-antiport. Magnesium leaves the cell in exchange for sodium.

It took us 25 years to learn the exact mechanism by which this operates. Only recently, in 2012, could we at last claim we have identified the gene that decides the amount of what we refer to as a "magnesium exchanger" in the cells. This is important because this sodium-magnesium exchanger is present in all cells in our body. It's the main magnesium efflux system. It's important to know that this system can become blocked by certain pharmacological substances, which inhibit the magnesium influx from the cell. One of the important functions of certain drugs is to keep magnesium in the cell. It was also found that this transporter might be genetically different in a subgroup of patients with Parkinsons disease, or might be differently regulated in conditions such as preeclampsia, as we have been able to show recently. Only now, knowing the genetic backgrounds of magnesium regulation, can more specific investigations into the contribution of this system to various diseases made.

Magnesium must be reabsorbed in the glomerulus and the kidneys. Most is absorbed in the thick ascending limb (TAL), but also in the distal convoluted tubule (DCT), with something like 90-95% being retrieved in one of these two ways. The mechanism for this retrieval is similar to the mechanism that enables magnesium reabsorption in the intestines. Again, we have a para-cellular pathway and we have trans-cellular pathways, which involve several different genes that regulate the influx of magnesium into the cell. A number of diseases are caused by inherited genetic defects. The human body has several magnesium transporters that regulate our magnesium status and hereditary defects in these magnesium transporters are known to cause some of these diseases.

On top of this, there is the question of whether people actually receive the ideal daily intake of something in the range of 300 to 420 milligrams of magnesium. Do most of us eat sufficient magnesium-rich foods? Nuts and seeds are rich in magnesium. So too are green vegetables and salads, which of course contain chlorophyll. In fact, everything that's green is full of magnesium because the green color comes from chlorophyll, in which magnesium is the central ion. If we remove magnesium from chlorophyll, it loses its color. While it's easy to diagnose a magnesium deficiency in plants precisely because they have a bleached appearance, it's not so easy in the case of humans. What a pity nature didn't make us green, like we once imagined inhabitants of Mars to be! Our work would have been so much easier.

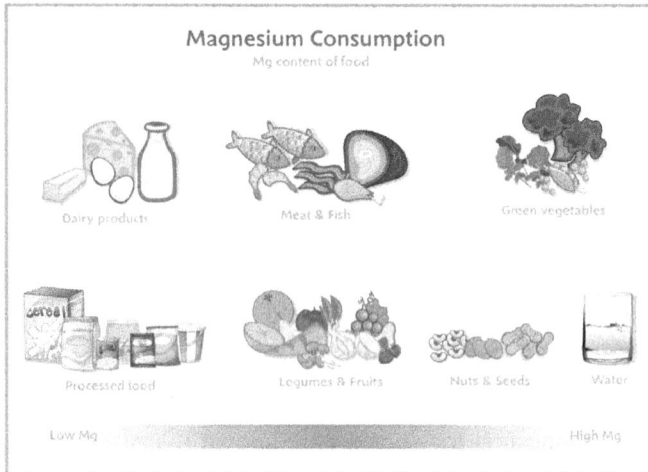

Figure 3: Magnesium Consumption

Processed foods are notoriously low in magnesium, since all processing of food diminishes the magnesium content. For instance, simply boiling a potato extracts 50% of the magnesium, which is lost in the cooking water. And what do we with the water? We usually throw it away. Today, of course, more and more of us are eating processed foods that contain little nutrition, and certainly little magnesium, so that magnesium deficiency is increasing.

In Australia, 50% of males and 40% of females obtain less than the recommended daily intake of magnesium. One study showed that the average intake was only 280 milligrams. Another study, this time conducted in 2008 in Germany, revealed that 26% of men and 28% of women have an intake of magnesium that's below the daily suggested requirement.

If we examine the data for the different age groups in the study, we discover that the incidence of low intake in females in their teens runs at 56%, double that of the average woman. One reason for this is that these are the years when young woman tend to indulge in dieting in an attempt to match up to Western society's stereotype of the ideal female body. It's also during the teen and young adult years that women tend to embark on pregnancy, with many of them starving themselves during the pregnancy to keep their figure, thereby greatly reducing their magnesium intake—a practice that's good for neither the mother nor the child.

Another German study from 1995 looked at the serum magnesium concentration. The threshold chosen in this study was extremely conservative, deeming females to be deficient in magnesium only if their level was below 0.67 mM. Today, a minimum level to maintain one's health is considered to be 0.75 mM, with 0.85 mM and above the optimum. By today's standards, the incidence of magnesium deficiency would be much higher. But even using the conservative levels of the 1995 study, a low plasma magnesium concentration was evident in about 10% of the population but the incidence was double in women age 18 to 24.

We encounter an additional problem as we age. We mentioned that our bones serve as our magnesium storehouse. We did a study that measured the magnesium concentration in the bones of traffic accident victims demonstrated that the older people become, the lower the magnesium content of their bones. When we are elderly, we don't have a good store of magnesium. We also lose our ability to release magnesium from our bones efficiently. Because the process takes longer, it becomes more difficult to maintain a consistent serum magnesium level.

Crucial to this whole picture is the fact that our acid-base affects our magnesium balance. One of our studies, some years ago now, determined the urinary net acid excretion as a parameter of an individual's acid-base status. What we see is that the higher the acid excretion, the higher the urinary magnesium loss. It is now known simply by aging we slide into a latent acidosis, due to reduced kidney function, which drives magnesium out of the body. This may be the reason the magnesium store in our bones decreases as our years mount.

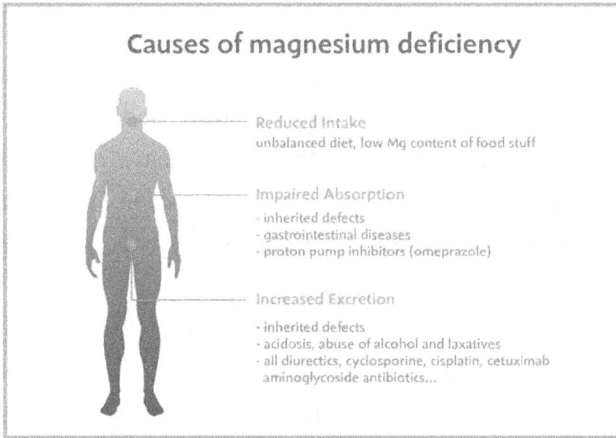

Figure 4: Causes of magnesium deficiency

Humans vary in their ability to absorb magnesium. Some have no difficulty with magnesium uptake, while others with a lower absorption capacity slip into a deficit much earlier in life. Part of this may be due to so-called polymorphisms of the genes involved in magnesium regulation. Tiny changes in efficacy of production of magnesium regulating systems might influence the ability of an individual to stay in balance. A variety of gastrointestinal diseases also play a part in reducing our ability to absorb magnesium. Generally, all diseases or infections leading to diarrhea will tremendously reduce the ability to absorb magnesium from the intestines. An often-overlooked side effect of proton pump inhibitors is to lower our ability to release magnesium from our food. Long-term intake of these proton pump inhibitors has been known to induce severe magnesium deficiency. These proton pump inhibitors reduce the production of gastric acid, and if we don't produce sufficient gastric acid, magnesium simply isn't released from food or from some supplements. Magnesium that isn't bioavailable is then excreted. Indeed, one of the most important factors in the induction of magnesium deficiency is increased excretion via the fecal or urinary route.

Alcohol also increases magnesium excretion, since alcohol is a diuretic. Alcohol abuse is a major cause of magnesium deficiency. Whenever you seen an alcoholic with shaky hands, the shaking is mainly due to a lack of magnesium. The smart thing is to drink less, while also increasing your magnesium intake. (Should you wish to visit Munich during Oktoberfest, you'd be wise to take plenty of magnesium before you imbibe. You'll certainly fare better the next day, since magnesium is an antidote to hangovers! But you do have to take it in advance to get the maximum benefit, as we can testify from experience.)

Many widely used drugs influence kidney function. Diuretics, whether they are potassium sparing or not, influence magnesium status. Increased diuresis itself drives magnesium out of the body. Cyclosporine, a substance all transplant patients must take the rest of their lives, is an extremely strong inhibitor of the magnesium reuptake systems in the kidneys, which is particularly poignant since all transplant patients need high doses of magnesium (though unfortunately they don't get the right amount, as most doctors are unaware of this). The same is

18

true of cancer therapies such as Cisplatin and Cetuximab, both of which are used especially in colon cancer therapy but induce dramatic magnesium deficits by inhibiting reabsorption in the kidneys. Antibiotics, especially aminoglycoside antibiotics, also inhibit reuptake of magnesium in the kidneys. Consequently, all patients taking these antibiotics require magnesium supplementation.

We have covered the problem of gastrointestinal malabsorption, but there are also endocrine causes of hypomagnesemia. (When we speak of too low a plasma-magnesium concentration, keep in mind that plasma and serum are the same thing when it comes to magnesium, as we pointed out earlier.)

Another cause of magnesium deficiency is stress. Stress will induce cellular magnesium losses, leading to a short-lived increase in plasma magnesium concentration. This increase will be normalized by increased urinary excretion, however, the reuptake of intracellular magnesium will reduce plasma magnesium and at the end a magnesium deficit remains. Long-lasting stressful periods are therefore a major cause of magnesium deficiency, as long as reasonable magnesium supplementation doesn't keep up with the losses.

Excessive sweating can also lead to significant loss, which is why athletes are smart to take magnesium in their sport. However, the content of magnesium in sweat decreases if we sweat a lot. For instance, soccer players lose more magnesium when they start training than when they are in a trained phase. Nevertheless, it's important to realize that we lose significant amounts of magnesium when we sweat, and take steps to replace it. But note that magnesium supplements should be taken in the regeneration phase and not directly before a competition. Too much magnesium could slow down the reaction phase somewhat (which you don't want when running a 100 meter sprint) or induce some softening of stool (which is also not very pleasant when running a marathon, for example).

6

How to Recognize Magnesium Deficiency

What are the main symptoms of magnesium deficiency? Unfortunately, there's no single obvious symptom. It's not as simple as saying, "I have a cramp." If you have a cramp, it's likely you do have a deficiency, but that's far from the most important symptom of a deficiency.

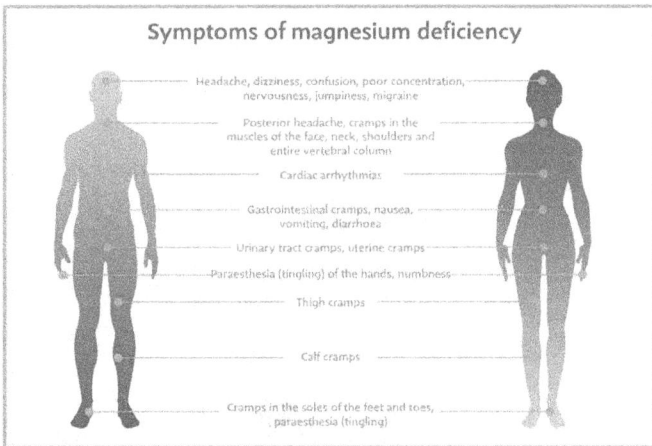

Figure 5: Symptoms of magnesium deficiency

Magnesium deficiency can result in headaches, dizziness, nervousness, confusion, poor concentration, migraines, and cramp in the muscles of the face, neck, shoulders, and the entire vertebral column. Indeed, cramps anywhere in the body can be connected to a deficiency of magnesium. But adequate magnesium isn't only a means of avoiding such things as calf cramps. Rather, it's truly essential for life. The fact is, because a magnesium deficiency is related to many diseases, it manifests in quite a variety of symptoms.

Having said there are no obvious indicators, we should add that a high percentage of cardiac arrhythmias are due to magnesium deficiency. Another small but strong indicator of a deficiency is tingling of the eyelid. If you find your eyelid tingling, you can assume your magnesium is low, and doctors are wise to watch for this in patients.

The majority of medical patients are hypomagnesemic (have low serum magnesium concentration)—although the condition isn't generally identified because doctors don't tend to test for this, since it's not currently part of the clinical routine. Despite the lack of testing, studies show that only a minority of patients whose magnesium status is tested fall within the optimal range of concentration, which is 0.85 to 1.1 mmol per liter. Only a tiny number have higher values. Again, the clinical signs of hypomagnesemia are nonspecific and can show up either in the neuromuscular area, the central nervous system, the metabolic system, or especially the cardiovascular system.

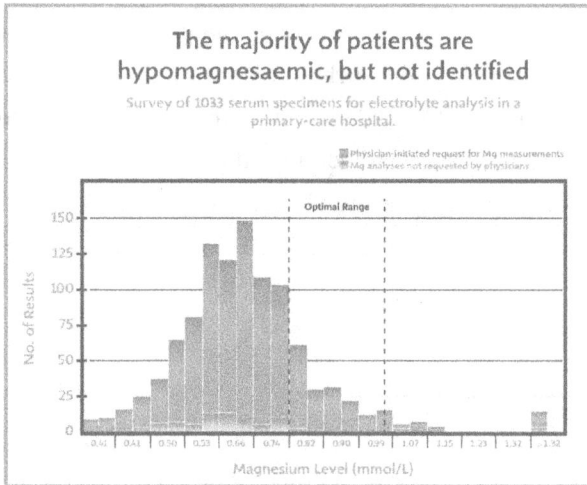

Figure 6: The majority of patients are hypomagnesaemic

We have very convincing data on the importance of magnesium for the cardiovascular system. In a small yet poignant study, fourteen women received a diet with only 100 milligrams of magnesium for up to 78 days to induce magnesium deficiency in the subjects. Since this is generally unethical, it wasn't easy to get the study approved by the ethical committees. The FDA in the United States ultimately sanctioned it, since the point was that if 25% of the American population eats only about 100 milligrams of magnesium on a daily basis, we should be able to duplicate the effects in a clinical setting and see what the effects may be.

The fourteen women selected for the study were closely monitored. In five of them, severe cardiac arrhythmias occurred. Of course, when the arrhythmias were detected, magnesium supplementation was administered, and the arrhythmias disappeared. None of the women experienced a cramp in their calf, yet a third of them experienced cardiac arrhythmias, which confirms that arrhythmia is a good indicator of a magnesium deficiency.

7

Your Heart and Brain Are at Risk

We can treat cardiac arrhythmias with magnesium supplementation. In fact, we have seen from studies how oral magnesium supplementation has the same effect as a magnesium infusion through the blood in terms of resumption of a normal cardiac rhythm in patients undergoing cardiac surgery. Surprisingly, oral supplementation has even shown itself to be somewhat superior. Since the reduction of arrhythmias can be accomplished at least as effectively with oral doses of magnesium as with intravenous infusion, this simplifies treatment.

Similarly, we have seen in studies of both men and women that there's a significant correlation between decreased plasma magnesium concentration and the risk of sudden cardiac death. Quite simply, we can avoid up to three quarters of sudden cardiac deaths by ensuring an individual has the correct concentration of magnesium. In other words, in some cases your magnesium status literally determines whether you live or die of sudden cardiac failure.

In a recent study from Germany, 4,000 individuals were followed over a period of twelve years. The subjects were divided into two groups according to their plasma magnesium concentration, with the split determined by those above 0.73 mmol per liter and those below. The group with the low magnesium concentration experienced a mortality rate significantly higher than the group with the higher concentration. Again, the evidence shows that magnesium is a determining factor in how long you live.

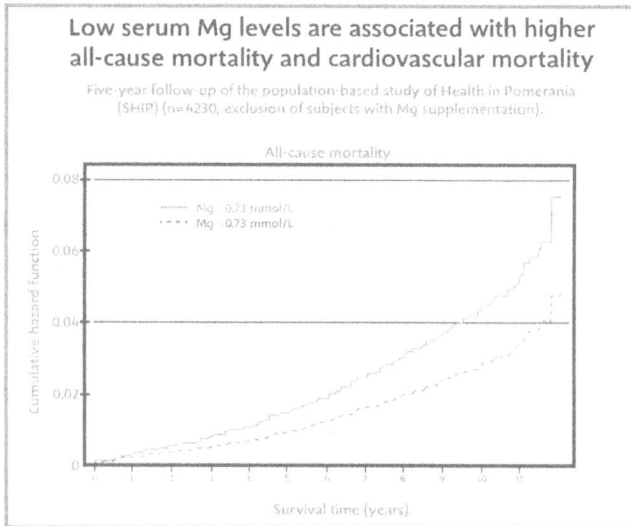

Figure 7: Low serum magnesium levels are associated with higher all-cause mortality and cardiovascular mortality

Magnesium status is also inversely associated with the risk of stroke. Studies have shown that you can reduce your risk of stroke by about 50% by having an appropriate concentration of magnesium in your body. Indeed, in a meta-analysis of prospective studies it was found that an increase of 100 milligrams of magnesium per day results in a 10% decrease in the risk of stroke.

The fact is, magnesium also greatly reduces the occurrence of atherosclerosis. The higher the concentration of magnesium in the body, the lower the risk of any form of coronary heart disease. As a recently published meta-analysis revealed, in the vast majority of studies that were considered, increased serum magnesium concentrations resulted in a reduction in risk of total cardiovascular events. Only a small number of studies failed to reflect this, in contrast to the overwhelming majority of studies. This is extremely important, given that the majority of us fall into the sector of the population in which serum magnesium concentrations are relatively low. In particular, women can avoid nearly two-thirds of all cardiovascular disease, though the percentage isn't quite as high in males. Women especially profit from a high plasma magnesium concentration.

Another recent and rather large study of the correlation of dietary magnesium and plasma magnesium concentration and the risk of coronary heart disease followed 86,000 women for up to 28 years. The data shows that there is only a small risk reduction with increased magnesium intake if you look at the incidence of total cardiovascular events. However, if you differentiate into non-fatal and fatal coronary heart disease, there is a stunning result. Non-fatal heart disease is nearly uninfluenced by increased magnesium intake, whereas there is a clear and significant negative correlation of increased magnesium intake with fatal heart disease in this population of women. This result simply shows that it is your magnesium status that decides whether you survive a cardiac attack. So it's a wise idea to avoid a magnesium deficit whenever you can—something that isn't too complicated, as we will see later.

There are now many studies of large numbers of people that show the change of relative risk of cardiovascular disease if you have, for instance, 0.2 mmol per liter higher plasma magnesium. You can reduce your cardiovascular disease risk by 30% simply by increasing your level of circulating magnesium. In the case of ischemic heart disease, there is a risk reduction of 17% when magnesium circulating in the blood is high, with a whopping 40% less cases of fatality in the case of ischemic heart attacks.

In other words, the higher your magnesium intake, the lower your risk of acquiring coronary heart disease, and the greater your chances of surviving a heart attack if you are unfortunately enough to experience one. This is just further evidence that, as a general health practice, we should aim to ensure a high plasma magnesium concentration in the entire population—the higher, the better.

In the case of coronary heart disease, using magnesium to treat patients can greatly reduce the need for other treatments such as calcium channel blockers, beta blockers, and nitrates. Indeed, we find supplementing a patient's magnesium to be extremely effective when it comes to their overall functionality.

8

Magnesium and Diabetes

Many diabetics have reduced magnesium content in their serum. In fact, the incidence of hypomagnesemia in type two diabetics is much higher than in their healthy counterparts. The reason is that diabetics have polyuria and simply lose a lot of magnesium.

Magnesium is also closely related to the risk of becoming diabetic in the first place. The higher the daily magnesium intake, the lower the risk of developing diabetes. For instance, in a meta-analysis of seven prospective cohort studies with over 600,000 subjects involved, about a 15% reduction of risk with each 100-milligram increase in daily intake of magnesium was found.

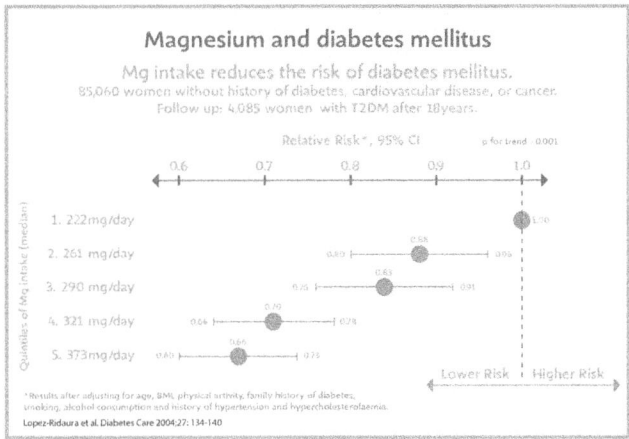

Figure 8: Magnesium and diabetes mellitus

So, magnesium is extremely protective against developing type two diabetes. This was also shown in a study by a friend of ours in Mexico, Professor Fernando Guerrero-Romero, who along with others conducted a 10-year follow-up study on plasma magnesium concentration in the population and correlated it with the percentage of the population who developed diabetes mellitus. The lower the plasma concentration, the higher the risk of becoming diabetic up to a factor of five. What we also see from this study is that if you have a high plasma magnesium concentration, you can just about completely avoid the risk of developing diabetes.

Another large epidemiological study, the already mentioned Nurses Health Study, demonstrated that a large increase of magnesium resulted in a significant reduction in the risk of diabetes, up to some 40%.

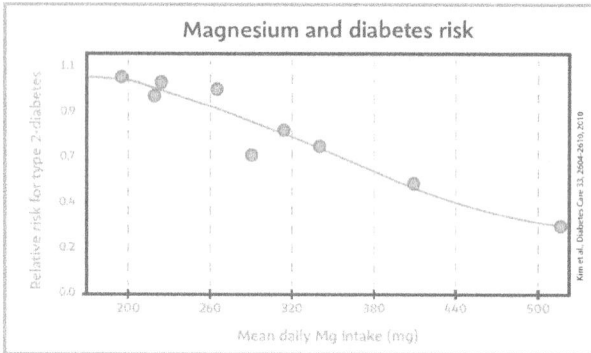

Figure 9: Magnesium and diabetes risk

A recent study out of Australia (by Simmons, Joshi, and Shaw) contrasts those who don't take antihypertensive medication with those who do. Patients on antihypertensives have seven times more often hypomagnesemia than controls. In comparison to these normal healthy adults, patients newly diagnosed as diabetic have an even higher incidence of hypomagnesemia which increases by a factor of ten.

A meta-analysis of studies involving several hundred thousand people also show that the relative risk of developing diabetes is significantly reduced by increased magnesium intake. For instance, with only a 100 milligram daily increase, the risk goes down by 15%. This is a very small increase in magnesium intake, and greater quantities decrease the risk considerably more effectively.

In our professional opinion, we would say that by doubling your intake of magnesium you can reduce your relative risk by 50%.

What's the chemistry behind this? During recent years, much has been learned on this subject.

Magnesium significantly influences the insulin status and the function of insulin in our bodies. In patients with hypomagnesemia, we find diminished glucose transport capacity as the sensitivity of the insulin receptor is established by sufficient magnesium. But also insulin secretion is below normal. Additionally, we find impairment in the post-receptor insulin signaling cascade. In sum, what happens intracellularly when insulin works on a cell is intensively influenced by the individual's magnesium status.

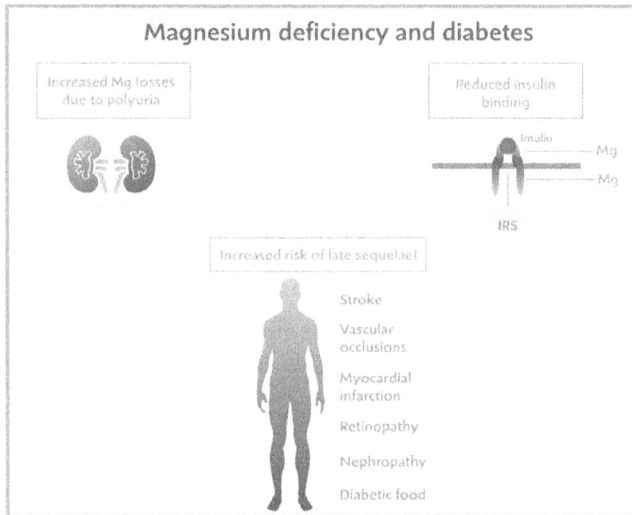

Figure 10: Magnesium deficiency and diabetes

A study of oral magnesium supplementation in elderly diabetic patients, especially focusing on their vascular function, resulted in a dramatic increase in flow-mediated dilation in the magnesium supplemented group. This is a good parameter for the overall functioning of the vasculature. In the control group, there was no change from the baseline after a month. This leads us to conclude that high-dose magnesium supplementation has a positive effect on vascular health in diabetics. This makes sense, given that the problems with diabetics relate mainly to blood flow through the organs and the late complications that result in these patients. We have clear evidence that the system can be significantly improved with proper magnesium supplementation.

Also, pre-diabetic patients—those with metabolic syndrome—benefitted from daily magnesium supplementation. A study was done in Mexico by the already-mentioned group with which we are cooperating intensively. This was a randomized, double-blind, placebo-controlled study. From it, we see that when pre-diabetics receive high doses of magnesium, glucose goes down—especially hemoglobin A1C, which is a clinically relevant effect. The capacity to produce insulin is also improved, and the HOMA-IR index goes down—a considerably improved situation.

We need to mention that patients received 2.5 grams of magnesium chloride per day. You might wonder why magnesium chloride was used. Well, it was the only type of magnesium available in Mexico at that time. Although it's not the ideal, it nevertheless worked. The dose was high, delivering 600 milligrams of magnesium. The problem is that it tastes horrible! Once you taste magnesium chloride, you're unlikely to take it for long.

We are currently doing a number of studies with the same Mexican researchers, at The Institute of Diabetes Research. In the newer studies, we have exchanged magnesium chloride for magnesium citrate. Magnesium citrate tastes better, which increases compliance. There's another factor that comes into play with magnesium chloride: it induces a state of acidosis in the body. Whenever a person takes either magnesium chloride or calcium chloride, they induce acidosis. Hence neither of these are the optimal delivery method for magnesium supplementation. In contrast, magnesium citrate is an alkalizing substance, which benefits the body in a variety of ways. This is extremely important particularly for diabetics, as they often develop acute acidosis. With proper magnesium supplementation, a person can avoid hypomagnesemia as well as acidosis.

When looking at meta-analyses, we have to be cautious in drawing definite conclusions, since there are studies that show a positive effect and others that don´t. However, when we examine the studies in detail, we find those that showed a negative effect were studies in which magnesium preparations that aren't well absorbed were used. The dosage was also extremely low. A failure to compare apples with apples and oranges with oranges is frequently a problem with studies. It's crucial to compare things that offer a legitimate comparison, both in the type of substance used and the dosage. In the case of those studies that show supplementation to be extremely effective, all used high doses of the optimum form of magnesium. So it's extremely important which kind of magnesium salt is used, and of course in what dosage.

We need to mention one other study from the same group in Mexico, because it addresses what we believe to be a common problem—diabetics who also suffer from depression. In this study, one group took magnesium, while the other group took the antidepressant Imipramine. The antidepressant clearly worked, with the depression score falling from 16 to around 11 on the scale. However, and this is something that was quite surprising, magnesium supplementation proved to be just as effective.

A factor we must consider is that we were able to show a long time ago that Imipramine inhibits the efflux of magnesium from the cells. Especially if this happens in neural cells, the intracellular magnesium levels stay high. So even in the case of the antidepressant, magnesium is involved. But the great news is that a sufficiently high dose of magnesium can achieve the same effect without any of the side effects with which long-term intake of this antidepressant drug is often connected.

The main point of this study is that magnesium obviously has a fundamental effect on the nervous system. One of its most important functions is to physiologically block the NMDA receptor, which has a magnesium binding site that's in equilibrium with magnesium outside the cells. The higher our magnesium intake, and the higher our plasma magnesium concentration, the more the receptor is blocked.

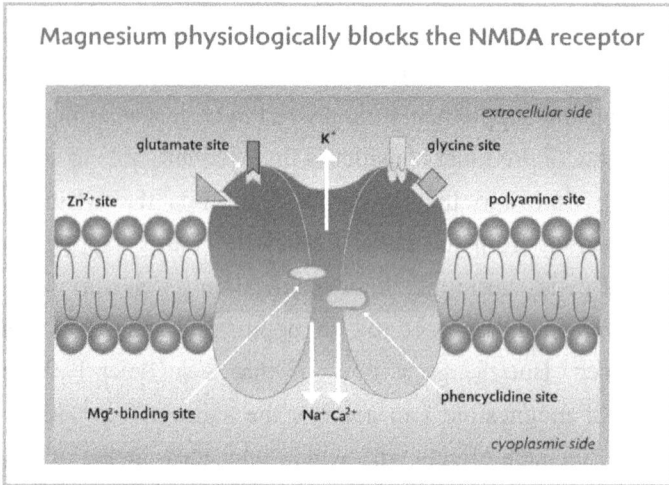

Figure 11: Magnesium physiologically blocks the NMDA receptor

Of course, we don't want the receptor to be completely blocked, since an over-excitation of this receptor isn't beneficial to us. For example, we require low activity in these receptors for learning and memory. Though we so far don't have human studies on this, a study from animal experiments is illuminating. These animals received either a normal diet of magnesium or a magnesium-deficient diet. The learning and memory capability was much lower in the magnesium-deficient group.

[9]

Magnesium and Neurological Issues

A recent discovery concerns magnesium and Alzheimer's disease. In patients with Alzheimer's, the ionized magnesium levels in plasma are reduced. We also know that the trafficking and processing of the amyloid-beta protein responsible for the problems associated with Alzheimer's is significantly influenced by magnesium. When there is a magnesium deficiency, this protein precipitates much earlier than with higher concentrations of magnesium. Also, low serum magnesium levels correlate with clinical deterioration in Alzheimer's disease. By avoiding low magnesium intake (and acidosis, of course), we give ourselves some protection against this devastating disease.

Another important area in which magnesium plays an important role is Parkinson's disease. In Germany alone, some 300,000 people suffer from Parkinson's today. This represents a dramatic increase in recent years. But how might magnesium help? It's known that magnesium in vitro has both preventive and ameliorating effects in rats.

It's also known that certain genes contains genetic variants in Parkinson's disease patients. One of these genes is the SLC41A1 gene, which as we can show encodes for the sodium-magnesium exchanger. This system takes magnesium out of the cell. The problem with Parkinson's patients might be that they have a magnesium efflux that's more active than we find in individuals who don't have this genetic defect. We can speculate that Parkinson's is connected to a change in the intracellular magnesium homeostasis. We are just now inaugurating clinical studies financed from the Michael J. Fox Foundation on magnesium treatment in Parkinson's patients. It's only two or three years ago that no one knew there's a connection between magnesium sensitive genes and Parkinson's disease.

Another neurological issue is the problem of headaches, especially migraines. We have known for some time that the magnesium concentration in the plasma, blood cells, saliva, cerebrospinal fluid, and cerebral cortex is reduced in those who experience migraines. In one study, the intracellular ionized magnesium in the brain was measured using nuclear magnetic resonance, which is a fairly complex process and not something that can be done routinely. The concentration of magnesium was high in the control group, but low in the group suffering from migraines. Concerning different severities of migraines it was shown that the greater the severity of the migraine, the lower the free magnesium concentration in the brain.

A study using 600 milligrams of Magnesium Diasporal, a brand name pharmaceutical grade magnesium citrate often used in our studies, over a period of twelve weeks showed a significant reduction in the frequency of migraine attacks.

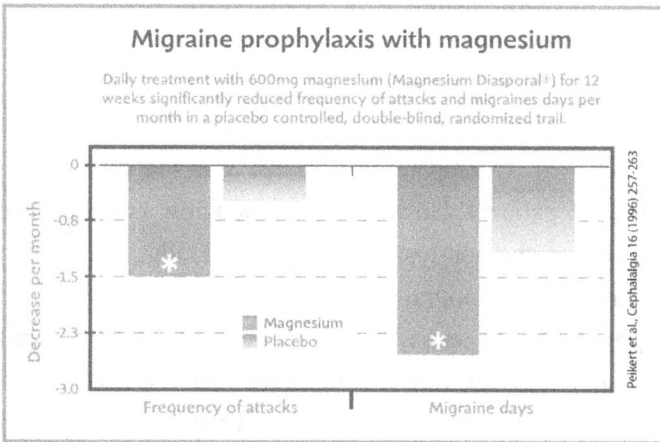

Figure 12: Migrain prophylaxis with magnesium

This study was later repeated, again using supplementation of 600 milligrams per day over twelve weeks. In the placebo group, there was no change in the intensity of pain. In contrast, in the group supplemented with magnesium the pain intensity was considerably reduced—in fact, almost halved.

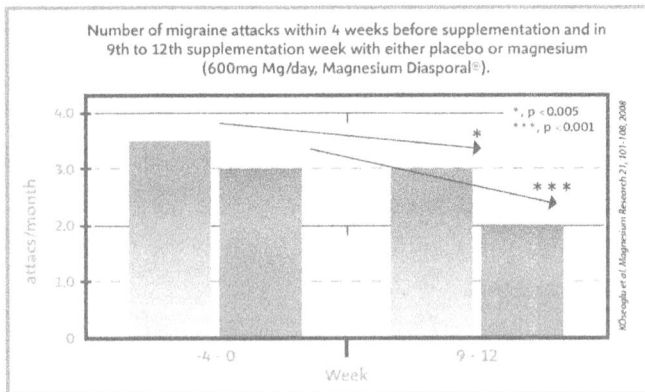

Figure 13: Migraine attacks

We wish to emphasize that this was the effect for a group of patients. However, we now know that we have responders and non-responders. It's generally the case that around 50% of migraine patients respond to magnesium supplementation extremely well, whereas others don't respond. We also want to emphasize that you need a high dose. Some subjects who experienced 600 milligrams with no effect were given higher doses. If 900 milligrams had no effect, we tried 1200 milligrams, which produced some effect. However, at 1500 milligrams the migraines were gone. It's a question of titrating the patient according to their specific need.

At these larger doses, we have to consider possible side effects. The only side effect that can occur is the loosening of stool to the point of causing diarrhea. It's therefore unwise to begin supplementation with too large a dose at once. For instance, we might start with 400 milligrams. Of course, for some with constipation, the loosening effect of magnesium is a welcome side effect. But about 10-15% of individuals will experience too much loosening at even 400 milligrams.

Thankfully, people tend to become accustomed to magnesium supplementation, which allows us to increase the dose. A person might begin on 400 milligrams, have no adverse reaction, and increase from there—in the case of someone whose migraines continue, perhaps going to 800 milligrams next, split over two doses at different times of day. If the person tolerates this amount, the dosage can be increased further if necessary.

When people can't tolerate more than 400 milligrams, there are two possible approaches. One is to add the second dosage only on alternate days, so that one day they receive 400 milligrams and the next 800 milligrams in two doses. The second is to dissolve the magnesium citrate in water and consume it over the course of the day, a sip at a time. Distributed throughout the waking day, the higher dosage becomes more tolerable. So if you find you have stomach or intestinal problems, sip your magnesium all day.

Patients with hereditary magnesium wasting need to take tremendously high amounts. Some require between 3,000 and 4,000 milligrams on a daily basis, which is the only way for them to remain in balance. Thankfully, genetically determined magnesium wasting is rare. The point is that patients' needs are all individual and need to be titrated accordingly.

A group at the New York Headache Center of Cornell University published a paper entitled "Why all migraine patients should be treated with magnesium." The paper suggests that deficiency is present in up to half of migraine sufferers and concludes that oral supplementation is warranted for all who experience migraines. In many cases this allows many patients to avoid taking medications that have severe side effects. Having mentioned side effects, we should add that the side effects of many drugs are significantly increased when magnesium concentrations are low. Many drugs reduce the capacity of the kidneys to reabsorb magnesium. A magnesium deficit is worsened in patients taking drugs, since many drugs work by increasing the calcium influx into the cells—an unwelcome side effect of such drugs. If magnesium concentrations are low, magnesium's ability to mitigate this situation is inhibited, which is how the side effects of the drugs can increase.

Magnesium is also effective in patients with tension headaches. In one study, 40 individuals from a special headache clinic, all of whom had suffered from tension headaches for years, consumed 600 milligrams of magnesium supplementation per day for two months. The results were dramatic, with some of them even becoming free of headaches.

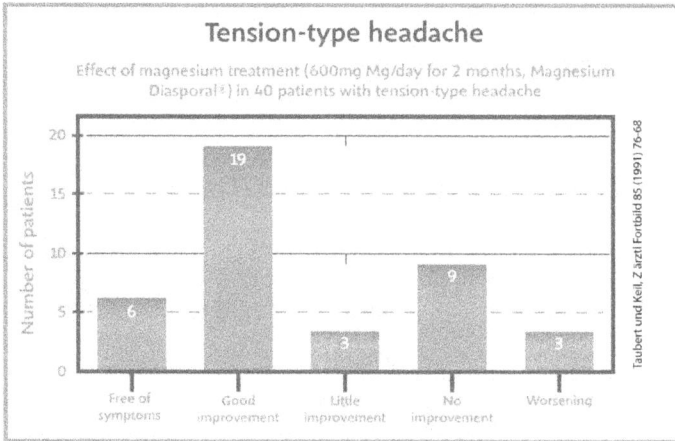

Figure 14: Tension headache

We need to emphasize that it can take two to three months to refill our magnesium stores, which of course are the bones. If the bone is tremendously depleted of magnesium, a significant increase in plasma magnesium concentration will only occur after some weeks of supplementation. Only then are we likely to see a reduction of headache attacks.

Magnesium is effective for asthma, too, relieving the bronchi. In a randomized crossover study with asthma patients who were treated orally with 400 milligrams of magnesium per day for three weeks, alongside a group who were given a placebo, the symptom index dropped significantly, with zero change in the placebo group. The use of a bronchial dilator also dropped significantly. Other studies done to the highest standards further confirm that magnesium makes a considerable difference.

[10]

Magnesium and Pregnancy

During the course of a pregnancy, there is a reduction of the concentration of plasma magnesium. In part this is connected to the dilution of the plasma, but also the need of the child as it's fed from the mother.

Reduced magnesium concentration during pregnancy has negative effects, some of which are serious. For instance, there's an increase in the rate of spontaneous abortion, as well as preterm births. We also see a reduced birth weight and impaired development of the fetus. In the mother, there can be pregnancy-induced hypertension, pre-eclampsia, and gestosis. The mother often also experiences frequent leg cramps and symptoms such as headaches, double or blurred vision, and abdominal pressure and nausea.

In a clinical trial involving 568 women, the group who received magnesium supplementation experienced a reduced number of days in hospital, less hemorrhaging, a reduction of premature labor from 8.2% to 2.8%, a lower number of cases of cervical insufficiency, and a slightly increased duration of pregnancy. The incidence of women experiencing premature labor was greatly reduced simply by supplementing with magnesium. There were also positive effects for the child, including a reduction in premature births, less need for intensive neonatal care, normalizing of birth weight, and increased body length. The total hospitalization in the magnesium group was significantly lower than for the placebo group.

Eclampsia is perhaps the most serious problem of pregnancy, connected to significant morbidity and mortality for both mother and child. Although the treatment of choice worldwide for eclampsia is magnesium infusion, sadly pregnant women don't receive oral magnesium supplementation on a global scale—with one exception, which is Germany, where more than two-thirds of pregnant women take magnesium.

Because of the high level of magnesium supplementation in Germany, which would have skewed our results, we conducted a study in Sweden, a country in which magnesium supplementation is largely unheard of. 60 women were part of the placebo-controlled study, all of them with an increased risk for pregnancy-induced hypertension. During the last three months of pregnancy, magnesium citrate was administered at a rate of 300 milligrams a day. Of 71 women who received no intervention, 18 experienced an increase of blood pressure. In the placebo group, 9 of the 29 candidates experienced increased hypertension. But in the group that received the magnesium, only 1 in 24 experienced an increase in blood pressure. We also measured the gene expression of various magnesium sensitive genes, which further revealed the effectiveness of this study.

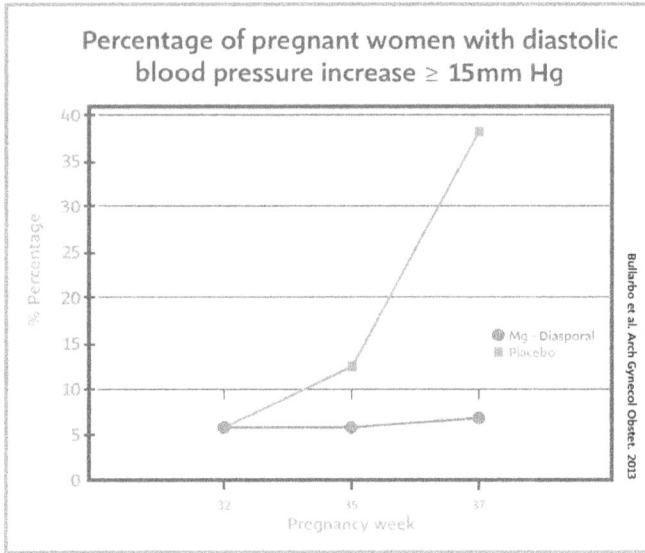

Figure 15: Percentage of pregnant women with diastolic blood pressure increase

Our intention now is to conduct a study of pregnant women in Sweden, Tanzania, Mexico, and China, which will allow us to investigate whether magnesium supplementation can significantly reduce pre-eclampsia, since this is such a serious issue. The incidence of pre-eclampsia in Sweden, where living conditions are extremely good, is very low at 3%. In Tanzania the incidence runs around 25%. China has an incidence of about 15% and Mexico around 20%. If we could avoid this problem, as the data so far indicates we can, it would be of tremendous benefit. It should also not be forgotten that excessive lactation during certain phases of breast feeding can result in a considerable loss of magnesium.

11

Other Benefits of Magnesium for Women

Magnesium can be used in women with dysmenorrhoea (painful menstruation, especially abdominal cramps). In an observational study of 64 women, high oral magnesium supplementation, at a rate of 600 milligrams a day, significantly improved the clinical symptoms of this affliction.

Another area in which magnesium has a positive effect is osteoporosis. Magnesium was used in a study to see if it could suppress bone turnover in postmenopausal osteoporotic women. In the control group, osteocalcin (which is a marker of bone turnover) remained more or less unchanged, whereas magnesium supplementation produced a positive increase. Bone degradation was also reduced in the magnesium group compared with the control group.

Magnesium is extremely important when it comes to osteoporosis, especially magnesium citrate. The citrate form not only assists us with absorbing magnesium, but also helps us avoid over-acidification, which is extremely detrimental to bone. By supplementing with magnesium citrate, we win on both counts.

12

When Magnesium Is the Wrong Thing to Give

Are there situations in which magnesium is contraindicated, even dangerous? For instance, should some individuals not be given magnesium supplementation?

There are people who have severe kidney dysfunction, and who therefore should avoid magnesium supplements. When a person is in stages four or five of chronic kidney disease, we find an increase in plasma magnesium concentration. In stages one, two, and three, there's no increase in concentration, even though the individual has a very low creatinine clearance. Generally, if you have a person with creatinine clearance above 30, there's no problem with magnesium supplementation. And, of course, we know who is in stages four and five, since they are already on dialysis. When someone is on dialysis, it's important to be extremely careful not to give magnesium without the oversight of a nephrologist. Having said this, for most of us magnesium is completely safe.

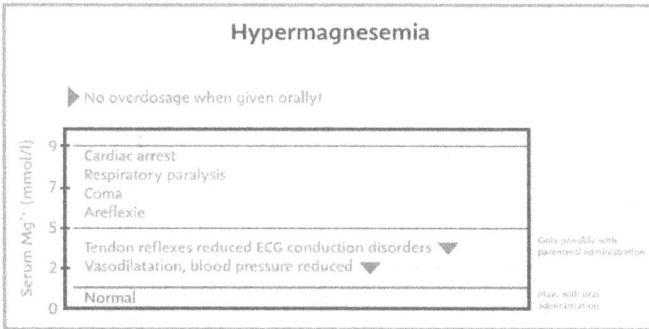

Figure 16: Hypermagnesia

If a person experiences hypermagnesemia, which is too much magnesium in the blood—such as up to 4 mmol per liter—there are effects, but these can only be triggered by mistakes in the administration of intravenous infusion of magnesium, never by oral administration. Such effects can take the form of areflexia (a lack of reflexes), respiratory paralysis, cardiac arrest, and coma. We would see the tendon reflexes reduced, ECG conduction disorders, and vasodilation resulting in reduced blood pressure.

When there is too much magnesium from oral administration, the surplus is excreted through the kidneys, which is a relatively easy task. In fact, it's more complicated for the kidney not to excrete the excess of magnesium. Even with supplementation of 1,000 or more milligrams, it's not possible to achieve more than 1.2 mmol per liter of blood.

13

Do You Have a Magnesium Deficiency?

How can you assess your magnesium status?

In the United States, Ronald J. Elin has done a lot of investigation of magnesium status utilizing methods employed in clinical chemistry. For instance, we can measure total serum magnesium concentration. We can also measure the serum ionized concentration, though this is a little more complicated. Additionally, we can use a 24-hour urine excretion method.

By far the easiest measurement to make is total serum concentration. An evidence-based reference interval for serum magnesium concentration has been established, where the lower limit is adjusted to a value that's healthy, which is 0.85 mmol per liter.

It's important to realize that a concentration above this figure still doesn't exclude magnesium deficiency, since the blood sampling procedure itself can sometimes induce a magnesium loss from the cells. This results because some people are anxious about having a needle inserted into their arm, and stress drives magnesium out of the cells. ATP is broken down, and bound magnesium is released and transported out of the cells, ending up in the plasma. So stress produces an artificial increase in our magnesium plasma concentration. Consequently, a person may have a serum magnesium concentration of 0.9 mmol per liter, which on the surface looks like they have no problem with a magnesium deficiency.

What this amounts to is that the serum concentration of magnesium is indicative when it's low, but it doesn't tell us anything if our levels appear normal or above normal. In fact, a study published by Yasmin Ismail, Abbas Isamil, and Adel Ismail advises that a health warning is needed for when there are "normal" results. This is to address the underestimated problem of using serum magnesium measurements to exclude magnesium deficiency in adults.

We want to quote from the conclusions of this study, published in Clinical Chemistry and Laboratory Medicine (48, 323-327, 2010), because the information is so important. The authors state, "The inaccuracy of serum magnesium as a biomarker of negative body stores, although well known among laboratorians, is not widely disseminated nor emphasised to clinicians. The perception that 'normal' serum magnesium excludes deficiency is not uncommon among clinicians, and this has contributed to underdiagnosis of chronic deficiency. Based on literature in the last two decades, magnesium deficiency remains common and undervalued, warranting a proactive approach by the laboratory because restoration of magnesium stores is simple, tolerable, inexpensive and can be clinically beneficial."

In addition to identifying low serum magnesium concentrations, it's important to observe clinical symptoms. As mentioned earlier, these can include such things as cardiac arrhythmia, cramps, migraine, and headaches. It's also important to identify risk factors for low magnesium intake by asking such questions as what the person eats and whether there are factors such as increased loss of magnesium—for instance, from use of a diuretic or a protein pump inhibitor. The simple reality is that a large percentage of people need magnesium supplementation.

How to Select the Best Magnesium Supplement

Which magnesium salt should be used for supplementation?

Studies have shown the superior efficacy of magnesium citrate, when compared for instance with amino acid chelate or magnesium oxide. When all three forms were administered at the same dosage, only magnesium citrate increased the magnesium plasma concentration. This was true both in a 24-hour study and in a 60-day study, both of which were based on supplementing with 300 milligrams of magnesium.

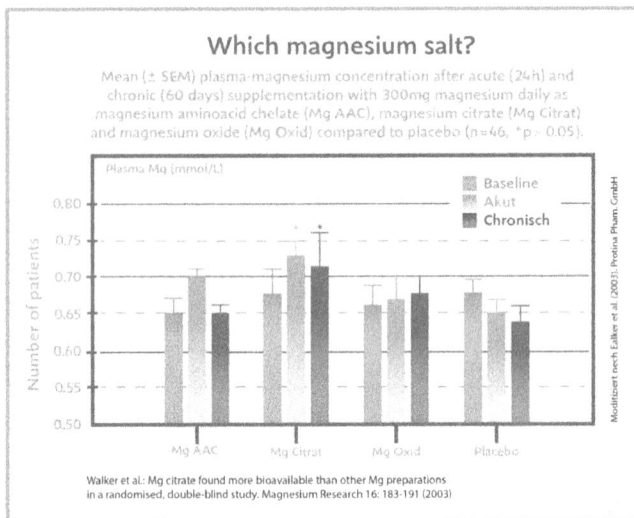

Figure 17: Which magnesium salt?

In another study using 600 milligrams of magnesium citrate, there was a significant advantage as the hours passed. In fact, serum magnesium levels increased for a period of twelve hours. In the placebo group, we see only the effects of the circadian rhythm, whereby magnesium levels are naturally lower in the morning but increase as the day goes on, reaching a peak in the evening. The time to give magnesium is therefore at night. We don't understand precisely why magnesium levels drop during the night, causing them to be low by morning, but suspect it has something to do with kidney function and hormone regulation.

This drop in plasma concentrations correlates with clinical symptoms. When do people tend to get leg cramps? Mostly at night and early in the morning. When do we tend to see myocardial infarction? There is a peak in the early morning hours. Arrhythmia also tends to occur at night. Such symptoms can be avoided simply by giving magnesium in the evening. One effect of the elevation and leveling out of plasma magnesium levels that this results in is that people sleep better because they are more relaxed. Incidentally, taken as a tablet, magnesium citrate isn't as effective, since it needs to be pre-dissolved to obtain the most value from it.

You might wonder whether you should take magnesium at the same time as calcium. My answer is an emphatic "no." If you put calcium and magnesium together, such as in pill form, the high magnesium inhibits the calcium uptake, and the high calcium inhibits the magnesium uptake. If calcium supplementation is necessary, there needs to be a period of several hours between ingesting the magnesium and the calcium. For example, you could take calcium in the morning and magnesium in the evening. Having said this, a normal diet usually contains adequate calcium for the average person in acid-base balance, so that there's no requirement for supplementation.

Of even great significance in terms of the effect of the kind of magnesium on the plasma magnesium concentration is the effect on the intracellular free

59

magnesium concentration in human leucocytes. When we supplement with magnesium oxide, there's only a small effect on the intracellular free magnesium concentration in the leucocytes, whereas there's a much larger effect when we use the citrate form. This is particularly significant because leucocytes are our immune cells, and a study published in Science in July 2013 shows that the level of magnesium in these cells is extremely important if they are to function effectively. Magnesium regulates the cytotoxic function of natural killer cells in patients with a defect in the MAGT1 transporter. This was also mentioned in the journal Nature, meaning that the significance of magnesium is now a serious matter for science.

Magnesium regulates antiviral immunity. The latest findings reveal the specific molecular function of free basal intracellular magnesium in eukaryotic cells. It's the intracellular free magnesium concentration in lymphocytes that's important, and we can show that with magnesium citrate we get a much better uptake than with magnesium oxide. Because of its impact on our immunity, magnesium deficiency has a truly negative effect and should be avoided.

We need to point out that this difference isn't something we can measure on a routine basis in everyday practice, since it's a complicated procedure requiring a magnesium-sensitive dye to load the cells—a process that takes quite a while. From such protocols, we know that only those who have a low magnesium plasma concentration register a major change, whereas those whose level is at or above 0.85 experience no change at all. However, we must emphasize that we find this increase not with magnesium oxide, only with magnesium citrate. A person with a relatively normal plasma concentration who would like to increase their level needs to use citrate. Since citrate is readily available, we might mention that it's highly desirable to have a plasma concentration that's as high as possible, since (as discussed earlier) this provides protection against sudden cardiac death, diabetes, and so on.

The point we are making about using citrate instead of other forms of magnesium is further borne out by the case of a child born with an error in the ability to reabsorb magnesium in the kidneys. The child developed severe cramps shortly after birth and was lucky to have a doctor who knew the importance of magnesium. Since this was a case of primary hypomagnesemia, it was initially treated intravenously. However, such treatment is neither practical nor desirable on a daily basis, so the child was then supplemented with the various forms of magnesium that are available. Those handling the case discovered that only with magnesium citrate were they able to establish the extremely high dose needed by the child—a dosage of 88 milligrams per kilogram of body weight. For a child weighing 20 kilograms, that's around 1,900 milligrams on a daily basis! Today, the child is still on the high dose of magnesium citrate and, at twelve or thirteen years of age, is symptom free.

What about other magnesium compounds, such as magnesium orotate? The problem with this form is that the actual amount of magnesium delivered is relatively low. Unfortunately, many preparations that contain this form don't state how much magnesium is supplied, only how much magnesium orotate is present. In such a case, you might get 500 milligrams of magnesium orotate, but only something like 30 milligrams of magnesium. Do you really want to take twenty tablets a day to get 600 milligrams?

Magnesium is only absorbed as an ion, not as a complex. Were it absorbed as a complex, the child I cited could easily be treated with a substance such as magnesium bisglycinate, which it's claimed is absorbed as a peptide. When magnesium is bound to something, it simply isn't absorbed. So it's not much better then magnesium oxide. The crucial issue with any supplement is an understanding of how it's transported into the cells.

When you are purchasing a magnesium product, be aware that just because something says "magnesium" doesn't mean it's useful to the body, since there are a number of factors involved in the absorption of the mineral. In its citrate form, it does the job—and you can take it lifelong. Professor Vormann has been taking it for more than 30 years.

Were magnesium absorbed into the cells through the skin, such as in the form magnesium oil, all we would need to do is go swimming in the ocean, since the ocean is high in magnesium. But magnesium isn't absorbed this way—although the oil can be used topically for certain skin diseases. The skin is nearly impermeable in the case of both magnesium and calcium. The genes now known to be involved in magnesium uptake all use only magnesium ions, not complexes. A wise decision therefore is to use magnesium citrate.

[15]

Conclusion

Even as earth's inhabitants migrated out of the original cradle of humanity, spreading out across the planet and colonizing continent after continent, so too the landmasses we now inhabit as a species have themselves shifted over eons of time. Land that was once submerged now forms mountains, while mountains were once the ocean floor. Vast regions have come into existence as a result of plate tectonics and volcanic activity that never existed before.

As humans spread out around the world, they encountered different climates producing different foodstuffs. Seasons came into play in a way they never had where our species had its nativity, hugely affecting the diet of our ancestors. Equally important, some of the younger soils produced not only different kinds but also different qualities of foods, since all growing media are not the same. Some zones were rich in one mineral but not in another, one nutrient but not another. And, too, in more recent times, modern farming methods have depleted soils in vast areas.

Today, we aren't often aware of how greatly the nutrients in our food supply vary according to how, where, and when the food was grown. With planes jetting fresh fruits to parts of the globe that don't naturally produce such fruit, and providing an abundance of meats, not to mention boatloads of foodstuffs shipped all over the world, it's easy to think of a Paleo diet in terms of the foods advocated for such a diet by books and websites that have made this their trademark. In reality a "paleo" diet consumed by our ancestors was considerably different from what we think of when we use this term today.

Yet there is a commonality among all these diets: their tendency to alkalinity and an abundance of health-giving organic minerals. Even when we do our best to eat a balanced diet, in our modern world we tend to shortchange ourselves when it comes to alkalinity and minerals such as magnesium.

The modern health-conscious individual is wise to select as alkalizing a diet as is practical, without neglecting an adequate supply of protein. Supplementation, especially when done under the supervision of a medical professional who is aware of the emerging science in the field, is a potent method of optimizing our health on many levels.

Never before has the science been available to guide us in riding ourselves of the scourge of magnesium-poor and acid-rich diets. As the facts become increasingly available, it's time for all of us, young and old, to take advantage of what we now know—and begin to experience a quality of life we didn't imagine possible, particularly as we age.

Appendix 1: Magnesium deficiency metabolic typing

For a very quick magnesium status indication it is recommended to go to:
www.magnesiumguide.com.au/magnesium-minute/

1. Magnesium Dietary Depleter (an issue with the intake of magnesium).

Description. A magnesium dietary depleter tends to have a diet lacking in whole grains, green vegetables, and legumes. According to a CSIRO study, approximately 50% of Australian men and 39% of Australian women are not getting sufficient magnesium in their diet. Such individuals respond well to both dietary changes and supplementation. It should be noted that absorption rises when dietary intake is low and drops when dietary intake, including supplements, is high. For example, a normal absorption rate for magnesium is 30-50%, though this can rise to 80% if intake is very low.

Assessment. You may be a magnesium dietary depleter if you complete the assessment in Table 1 with a score of less than 20.

• Magnesium Dietary Depleter Assesment Table
• Blood tests may or may not indicate deficiency, depending on severity.
- Plasma magnesium – low or on low side of normal. - Urinary magnesium – low or on low side of normal

Solution: Increase dietary sources of Mg and supplement with a highly bioavailable, clinically trialled Magnesium.

Dietary/Lifestyle. Increase consumption of organic wholegrains, green vegetables and legumes in the diet. Utilise Magnesium Rich Foods list from Bio-Practica.

Supplementation: Highly bioavailable, clinically trialed Magnesium. 1 sachet per day. Adjust dosing amount for children younger than 12yrs.

Table 1. Magnesium Dietary Depleter Assesment

How many times per week do you consume the following foods

Food	Almost everyday or everyday	Regularly (2-5 times per week)	Sometimes (once or less per week)	Rarely or never
Adzuki beans	3	2	1	0
Almonds (unsalted)	3	2	1	0
Baby beetroot leaves	3	2	1	0
Black-eyed peas	3	2	1	0
Beet greens	3	2	1	0
Brazil nuts (unsalted)	3	2	1	0
Brown rice	3	2	1	0
Buckwheat	3	2	1	0
Cashews (unsalted)	3	2	1	0
Figs	3	2	1	0
Halibut (fish)	3	2	1	0
Hazelnuts (unsalted)	3	2	1	0
Kelp	3	2	1	0
Kidney beans	3	2	1	0
Lentils	3	2	1	0
Linseeds	3	2	1	0
Low fat yoghurt	3	2	1	0
Macadamia nuts (unsalted)	3	2	1	0
Mixed lettuce greens (rocket, mesclun, endive, arugula, dandelion etc)	3	2	1	0
Millet	3	2	1	0
Oatmeal	3	2	1	0
Pecans (unsalted)	3	2	1	0
Pistachios	3	2	1	0
Pumpkin seeds	3	2	1	0
Rice bran/Oat bran/Wheat bran	3	2	1	0
Sesame seeds	3	2	1	0
Soy beans	3	2	1	0
Spinach or baby spinach	3	2	1	0
Spirulina	3	2	1	0
Sunflower seeds	3	2	1	0
Walnuts	3	2	1	0
SECTION 1. TOTAL SCORE				

A score less the 20 indicates a 'Dietary Depleter Type'   'Dietary Depleter Type' Yes ☐   No ☐

2: Malabsorber (organ issue: Intestines)

Description. Magnesium malabsorbers may be taking supplements and still not get results, or they may have to take higher than expected supplementation to produce results. Factors such as aging, poor digestion, high calcium levels, toxicity, and diarrhea can lead to ineffective absorption of magnesium. It is critical to supplement with a magnesium supplement that is well absorbed.

Assessment. The individual may experience symptoms of magnesium deficiency along with malabsorption issues such as nausea, vomiting, bloating, muscle wasting, unexplained weight loss, abdominal pain or cramping, bulky stools, steatorrhoea, undigested food in stool, and so on.

Tools for assessment:
Magnesium Malabsorber checklist Table 2
Practitioner Magnesium Malabsorber checklist
• Blood Tests: Magnesium may or may not be low depending on level of deficiency.
- Plasma Magnesium – low or low side of normal
- Urinary Magnesium – low or low side of normal
- RBC Magnesium (Reference range: 1.70-2.80 mmol/L)

A number of health conditions automatically indicate issues with magnesium absorption, including primary infantile hypomagnesaemia, ulcerative colitis, Whipples disease, short bowel syndrome, intestinal resection, and Crohn's disease.

Solution. Supplement with a highly bioavailable, clinically trialed magnesium, and address absorption issues.

Dietary/Lifestyle: In general, the degree of magnesium depletion correlates with the severity of diarrhea, stool fat content, and fecal magnesium concentration. The malabsorption of magnesium is secondary to formation of insoluble magnesium soaps, and a low fat diet improves magnesium balance in these patients. Other suggestions:
Repair and nourish the digestive tract using therapeutic agents such as glutamine and probiotics.
2. Calm and improve digestion with ginger, lemon juice, and water.
3. Add to the diet Slippery Elm powder, cook with cucumin, ginger and dill, to reduce inflammation and irritation to the GI lining.
4. Stop to eat, eat slowly, and chew well to ensure stimulation of natural digestion.
5. Reduce dietary phytates, oxalate, phosphorus and potassium if excessive as they reduce Mg absorption.

Supplementation:

Highly bioavailable, clinically trialed magnesium in a large bottle of water; drink throughout the day to maximise absorption. Adjust dosing amount for children younger than 12years.

Highly bioavailable curcumin extract to help reduce inflammation of the gastrointestinal tract.

High strength multi strain probiotic to support healthy gut microflora.

Gut healing formulations/support programs should be considered.

Genetics. Inherited mutation in the TRPM 6 gene – codes for an ion channel, resulting in defective carrier mediated transport of Mg in the small intestine. Absorption reduced from 70% to 35%. The defect can be overcome by increasing oral intake of magnesium to approximately 5 times that of normal daily requirements. Presents with hyocalcaemia, tetany, and seizures.

Table 2. Check list for Magnesium Malabsorber:

Signs and Symptoms
- 5 or more of the following signs and symptoms indicates a Mg Malabsorber type

Burps after meals regularly	☐
Heartburn regularly	☐
Flatulence regularly	☐
Bad breath regularly	☐
Takes Iron or Zinc supplements regularly without Magnesium	☐
Takes Calcium supplements without Magnesium	☐
Is over 50 years of age	☐
Regularly supplements their diet with protein powder (everyday)	☐
Eats a diet very high in protein (fish, chicken, eggs, meat) every day	☐
Has loose stools or diarrhoea 3 or more times per week	☐
Consumes a diet high in dairy products (more than 3 serves per day)	☐
Consumes a diet high in fatty foods daily (fried foods, butter, hamburgers, bacon, ice-cream, cheese, oils)	☐
Frequently has undigested food or fat in their stools (more than 3 times per week)	☐
Frequently uses antibiotics (more than 3 courses in the last 6 months)	☐
Has known low vitamin B1 levels	☐
Has known low vitamin D levels	☐
Has known low Vitamin B6 levels	☐
Has known high 'heavy metal' levels (Mercury, Cadmium, Lead, Aluminium, Arsenic)	☐
Has high 'Insulin' levels	☐
Has recent or known parasites or worms	☐
Steatorrhoea (excessive fats in the stool)	☐
Has unexplained weight loss	☐
Experiences abdominal pain or cramping	☐
Has some degree of intestinal permeability	☐

Known health conditions
- One or more of the following indications an Mg Malabsorber type

Irritable Bowel Syndrome (IBS)	☐
Hypoparathyroidism	☐
Crohn's disease	☐
Bulimia	☐
Ulcerative colitis	☐
Celiac disease	☐
Whipples disease	☐
Multiple Sclerosis	☐
Known genetic disorders affecting absorption (eg. TRPM 6 gene)	☐
Had intestinal resection	☐
Short Bowel Syndrome	☐
Medically diagnosed malnutrition	☐
Diabetes	☐

'Magnesium Malabsorber Type' Yes ☐ No ☐

72

3. Magnesium Hyper-excreter (organ issue: The kidneys)

Description. Hyper-excreters eliminate excessive amounts of magnesium through the kidneys and urine. They can often have normal levels of magnesium in blood tests, but what we are actually seeing is higher levels of magnesium being excreted and very little retained in the body. They will often have increased magnesium in the urine. It is critical to supplement with a magnesium supplement that gets into the cells and also address the issues that may be causing excessive excretion which can be dietary, drugs, kidney disorders, and so on.

Assessment. The individual may manifest symptoms of magnesium deficiency along with excretion issues such as kidney disorders, phosphate depletion, acidity, hypercalcaemia, and hormonal issues (PTH, calcitonin, antidiuretic hormone).

Tools for assessment:
• Magnesium Hyper-excreter checklist
Table 3
• Blood Tests: Magnesium may or may not be low depending on level of deficiency
- Plasma Magnesium – low or normal
- Urinary Magnesium – generally high or high side of

normal. - RBC Magnesium – (Reference range: 1.70-2.80 mmol/L)

A number of health conditions may automatically indicate excretion issues such as Barters syndrome, Gitelmans syndrome, primary hyperparathyroidism, malignant hypercalcaemia, hyperthyroidism, hyperaldosteronism, diabetes, etc.

Drugs such as diuretics, cytotoxic drugs (cisplatin, carboplatin, gallium nitrate), antimicrobial agents (aminoglycosides, antituberculous drugs, immunosuppressants), beta adrenergic agonists, amphotericin B, pentamidine, foscarnet, pamidronate, anascrin.

Osmotic diuretics such as mannitol and glucose cause marked increase in magnesium excretion.
[R Swaminathan, Magnesium Metabolism and its Disorders. Clin Biochem Rev. 2003 May; 24(2): 47–66.]

Solution. Dietary/Lifestyle: It is essential to reduce stress exposure, practice meditation and make the following dietary changes to avoid triggering excess excretion:
Reduce or avoid mannitol and glucose in the diet
Minimise carbonated drinks (fizzy drinks)
Reduce or avoid tea and coffee

Reduce or avoid alcohol

• Ensure you are drinking adequate water daily (8-10 glasses)

Supplementation:

1. Highly bioavailable, clinically trialed magnesium: 1-2 sachets per day, depending on severity of deficiency. Adjust dosing for children under 12 years.

2. Comprehensive Lymphatic Support Formula: To support kidney health.

3. Herbal calming formula: To reduce stress and the associated hormonal changes.

Table 3. Magnesium Hyper-excreter check list:

Consumes soft drinks / fizzy drinks daily	☐
Drinks 3 or more cups of coffee per day	☐
Drinks up to 5 cups of tea per day	☐
Consumes high sugar containing foods daily (chocolate, candy, lollies, ice-cream, cakes, biscuits, donuts etc.)	☐
Consumes fruit juice drinks everyday (two or more glasses of fruit juice per day)	☐
Lives or works in a high stress environment or is currently stressed	☐
Drinks alcohol everyday or more than 7 alcoholic drinks per week	☐
Does strenuous exercise or training more than 3 times per week (running, sports, gym etc)	☐
Experiences excessive sweating (more than 3 times per week)	☐
Takes steroid medication (e.g. Prednisolone, Symbacort, Cortisone)	☐
Takes Digitalis (Digoxin – a heart medication)	☐
Takes any of the following medication: Foscarnet (anti-viral drug), Amphotericin B (anti-fungal drug), Cyclosporin (immunosuppressant drug), Azathioprine (immunosuppressant drug), Cisplatin (chemotherapy drug).	☐
Has low Selenium levels	☐
Has high Calcium levels	☐
Has acid/alkali imbalance	☐
Has high Vitamin D	☐
Has high Potassium levels	☐
Has high blood pressure	☐
Has high Insulin levels	☐
Is often dehydrated (does not drink enough water)	☐

Known health conditions
- One or more of the following indications a Mg Hyper-excreter type

Alcoholism	☐
Chronic kidney disease (kidney failure, Dialysis)	☐
Genetic kidney disorder (eg. Barters syndrome, Gitelman syndrome)	☐
Diabetes	☐
Diabetic nephropathy	☐
Takes any kind of diuretic medication (Thiazides, Osmotic diuretics, Loop diuretics etc.)	☐
Nephritis	☐
Renal fibrosis	☐
Kidney stones	☐
Hyperparathyroidism	☐
Hyperaldosteronism	☐
Hyperthyroidism	☐
Hypocalcaemia	☐
Recurrent cystitis	☐
Recurrent kidney infections	☐

'Magnesium Hyper-excreter Type' Yes ☐   No ☐

4: Magnesium Demander (metabolic issue)

Description. The magnesium demander has an increased need for magnesium due to certain lifestyle factors. Those with increased demand include pregnant/lactating women, athletes, growing children, stressed individuals, and the aging.

Assessment. The individual may or may not initially manifest many symptoms of magnesium deficiency, but may have a health issue or condition that increases their body's metabolic need for magnesium.

Tools for assessment:
Magnesium Demander Checklist Table 4
Solutions.
Dietary/Lifestyle: Reduce stress and increase dietary intake of magnesium food groups.

Supplementation:
Highly bioavailable, clinically trialed magnesium: 1-2 sachets daily. Adjust dosing for children under 12 years.
Energy / Thyroid formula and or herbal calming formula - for highly stressed individuals.
Clinically Trialed Alkalising Mineral drink - for Athletes/high intensity exercise.

Table 4. Magnesium Demander check list:

Currently pregnant	☐
Recently pregnant (in the last 12 months)	☐
Breastfeeding or recently breastfed for longer than 12 months	☐
Recent traumatic stress, physical or emotional (in the last 6 months)	☐
Lives or works in a stressful environment or is currently stressed	☐
PMS or menstrual cramps	☐
Chronic lethargy or fatigue	☐
Has trouble sleeping most nights (more than 3 nights per week)	☐
Drinks alcohol everyday or more than 7 alcoholic drinks per week	☐
Over 50 years of age	☐
Strenuous exercise or training more than 3 times per week (running, sports, gym etc)	☐

**Known health conditions
– One or more of the following indicates an Mg Demander Type**

Insomnia	☐
Cardiovascular disease (Arrhythmia, Atherosclerosis, congestive heart failure or recent cardiovascular "event").	☐
High blood pressure	☐
Recent pancreatitis	☐
Recent blood transfusion	☐
Recent saline infusion	☐
Fibromyalgia	☐
Diabetes (insulin dependent)	☐
Osteoporosis	☐
PTSD (post traumatic stress disorder)	☐
Asthma	☐
An overactive thyroid, or underactive thyroid	☐
Depression	☐
Glaucoma	☐
Chronic headaches or migraines	☐
An endocrine condition such as Hyperaldosteronism or Hyperparathyroidism	☐
Have diagnosed Haemochromatosis (iron overload)	☐
In a previous pregnancy had high blood pressure or preeclampsia	☐
Taking oral contraceptives	☐
Recent severe burns	☐

'Magnesium Demander Type'   Yes ☐   No ☐

78

5. Magnesium Multi-depleter

Description. Any combination of low dietary intake, absorption, demand, and/or excretion issues. Such individuals often require magnesium supplementation and well as to have their multiple underlying issues addressed, according to which magnesium type issues they have. Having multiple depletion issues, magnesium status and underlying issues should be treated with high priority.

Assessment. The individual may evidence any of the above signs and symptoms of magnesium deficiency and/or known health conditions in any type.

Blood Tests:

- Plasma Magnesium – low
- Urinary Magnesium – low or high, depending on their types - RBC Magnesium – (Reference range: 1.70-2.80 mmol/L)

Solution.

Dietary/Lifestyle: Treat as for each individual type, as it presents. For example, an individual may present as multi-depleter; hyper-excreter/demander. Then treat as per these sections suggest.

Supplementation:

1. Highly bioavailable, clinically trialed Magnesium: 1-2 sachets daily or as prescribed depending on the severity of signs and symptoms. Adjust the dose for children under 12 years.

Appendix 2: YOUTUBE Video Resources:

MAGNESIUM DEFICIENCY QUESTIONS
ANSWERED BY PROFESSOR VORMANN:

Question 1: What are the factors to consider when selecting a Magnesium Supplement?
http://youtu.be/4RajrL8XMnM

Question 2: Which is best? Magnesium Tablet Vs Magnesium Powder: http://youtu.be/IbysEB2Zvw8

Question 3: What is your opinion of Multi Ingredient Magnesium Supplements?
http://youtu.be/pPPCmx39hjQ

Question 4: Is Magnesium Citrate the best form of Magnesium? http://youtu.be/zns3rr-ujXw

Question 5: Is Magnesium Citrate the best form of Magnesium? Long Answer.
http://youtu.be/nzqpiI7A7Es

Question 6: Is it true that Magnesium can be absorbed as a complex molecule? http://youtu.be/z-V0RbILlio

Question 7: Do we get enough Magnesium in our diet? http://youtu.be/_suUZzshxE0

Question 8: Is there a Magnesium Deficiency Crisis? Why? http://youtu.be/8yknNBC8azQ

Question 9: Can we deplete our Magnesium Levels?
http://youtu.be/vk-lQGjF8hA

Question 10: Why are high doses of Magnesium required? http://youtu.be/5ww7Pre586s

Question 11: Are there disease States that respond to high doses of Magnesium?
http://youtu.be/__RosCSP2UE

Question 12: Is there interesting research of the relationship of Magnesium status and Diabetes?
http://youtu.be/t2RxSsJdxdU

Question 13: How do you know how much available Magnesium is in a supplement?
http://youtu.be/u4KbqinKLJA

Question 14: Why is Magnesium essential during Pregnancy? http://youtu.be/CCEb1-u1fN0

Question 15: Why is Magnesium essential during Stress? http://youtu.be/AyqYWXDlRiU

Question 16: After 30 years of research into Magnesium in your opinion how important is Magnesium to health? http://youtu.be/PbkFRJPOeFQ

Question 17: When is the best time to take Magnesium? http://youtu.be/POUOgFFuhWk

Question 18: What is the relationship of Magnesium status and sudden cardiac death?
http://youtu.be/IWR-QmS7eo8

Question 19: What does the research tell us about Magnesium status and Cardiac disease?
http://youtu.be/Tf8YPUHxpUw

Bibliography

Vormann J. Magnesium In: Biochemical, Physiological, and Molecular Aspects of Human Nutrition, 3rd Edition Edited by: Stipanuk MH, Caudill MA. 747-758 Elsevier, 2012

de Baaij et al. **Regulation of magnesium balance: lessons learned from human genetic disease.** Clin Kidney J. 5: i15-i24, 2012

Nationale Verzehrs Studie II, Max Rubner Institut, BFEL, 2008

Kohlmeier et al. Versorgung Erwachsener mit Mineralstoffen und Spurenelementen in der Bundesrepublik Deutschland. In: Kübler, W., Andersen, H. J., Heeschen, W. (Hrsg.) Vera-Schriftenreihe Band V, Wissenschaftlicher Fachverlag Dr. Fleck, Niederkleen, 1995.

Rylander et al. Acid-base status affects renal magnesium losses in healthy, elderly persons. J Nutr. 136: 2374-7, 2006

Lameris et al. Drug-induced alterations in Mg2+ homoeostasis. Clin Sci. 123:1-14, 2012

Seelig MS. Consequences of magnesium deficiency on the enhancement of stress reactions; preventive and therapeutic implications. J Am Coll Nutr. 13: 429-46, 1994

Whang and Ryder. Frequency of hypomagnesemia and hypermagnesemia. Requested vs routine. JAMA 263:3063–4, 1990

Reffelmann et al. Low serum magnesium concentrations predict cardiovascular and all-cause mortality. Atherosclerosis 219:280-4, 2011

Larsson et al. Dietary magnesium intake and risk of stroke: a meta-analysis of prospective studies. Am J Clin Nutr. 95:362-6, 2012

Chiuve et al. Plasma and dietary magnesium and risk of sudden cardiac death in women. Am J Clin Nutr. 93:253-60, 2011

Chiuve et al. Dietary and plasma magnesium and risk of coronary heart disease among women. J Am Heart Assoc. 18; 2:e000114, 2013

Kim et al. Magnesium intake in relation to systemic inflammation, insulin resistance, and the incidence of diabetes. Diabetes Care 33:2604-10, 2010

Dong et al. Magnesium intake and risk of type 2 diabetes: meta-analysis of prospective cohort studies. Diabetes Care 34:2116-22, 2011

Guerrero-Romero and Rodríguez-Morán. Hypomagnesemia, oxidative stress, inflammation, and metabolic syndrome. Diabetes Metab Res Rev. 22:471-6, 2006

Simmons et al. Hypomagnesaemia is associated with diabetes: Not pre-diabetes, obesity or the metabolic syndrome. Diabetes Res Clin Pract. 87:261-6, 2010

Lopez-Ridaura et al. Magnesium intake and risk of type 2 diabetes in men and women. Diabetes Care 27:134-40, 2004

Larsson and Wolk. Magnesium intake and risk of type 2 diabetes: a meta-analysis. J Intern Med. 262:208-14, 2007

Barbagallo et al. Oral magnesium supplementation improves vascular function in elderly diabetic patients. Magnes Res. 23:131-7, 2010

Guerrero-Romero et al. Oral magnesium supplementation improves insulin sensitivity in non-diabetic subjects with insulin resistance. A double-blind placebo-controlled randomized trial. Diabetes Metab. 30:253-8, 2004

Barragán-Rodríguez et al. Efficacy and safety of oral magnesium supplementation in the treatment of depression in the elderly with type 2 diabetes: a randomized, equivalent trial. Magnes Res. 21:218-23, 2008

Barbagallo et al. Mg is reduced in mild-to-moderate Alzheimer's disease. Magnes Res. 24:115-21, 2011

Cilliler et al. Low serum magnesium level correlates to clinical deterioration in Alzheimer's disease. Gerontology 53:419-22, 2007

Yu et al. Magnesium modulates amyloid-beta protein precursor trafficking and processing. J Alzheimers Dis. 20:1091-106, 2010

Hashimoto et al. Magnesium exerts both preventive and ameliorating effects in an in vitro rat Parkinson disease model. Brain Res. 1197:143-51, 2008

Yan et al. Genetic variants in the RAB7L1 and SLC41A1 genes of the PARK16 locus in Chinese Parkinson's disease patients. Int J Neurosci. 121:632-6, 2011

Lodi et al. Deficient energy metabolism is associated with low free magnesium in the brains of patients with migraine and cluster headache. Brain Res Bull. 54:437-41, 2001

Peikert et al. Prophylaxis of migraine with oral magnesium: results from a prospective, multi-center, placebo-controlled and double-blind randomized study. Cephalalgia 16:257-63, 1996

Köseoglu et al. The effects of magnesium prophylaxis in migraine without aura. Magnes Res. 21:101-8, 2008

Mauskop and Varughese. Why all migraine patients should be treated with magnesium. J Neural Transm. 119:575-9, 2012

Taubert and Keil. Pilotstudie zur Magnesiumtherapie bei Migräne und Spannungskopfschmerz. Z ärztl Fortbild. 85, 76-68, 1991

Spätling and Spätling. Magnesium supplementation in pregnancy. A double-blind study. Br J Obstet Gynaecol. 95:120-5, 1988

Bullarbo et al. Magnesium supplementation to prevent high blood pressure in pregnancy: a randomised placebo control trial. Arch Gynecol Obstet. 288:1269-74, 2013

Wilimzig and Pannewig. High-dose oral magnesium
therapy in pregnancy. Der Allgemeinarzt 18:1466-71,
1994

Coburn et al. The physicochemical state and renal
handling of divalent ions in chronic renal failure. Arch
Intern Med. 124:302-11, 1969

Elin RJ. Assessment of magnesium status for diagnosis
and therapy. Magnes Res. 23:194-8. 2010

Ismail et al. The underestimated problem of using serum
magnesium measurements to exclude magnesium
deficiency in adults; a health warning is needed for
"normal" results. Clin Chem Lab Med. 48:323-7, 2010

Walker et al. Mg citrate found more bioavailable than
other Mg preparations in a randomised, double-blind
study. Magnes Res. 16:183-91, 2003

Wilimzig et al. Increase in magnesium plasma level after
orally administered trimagnesium dicitrate. Eur J Clin
Pharmacol. 49:317-23, 1996

Nestler et al. Magnesium Supplementation acutely affects
intracellular Mg^{2+} in Human Leukocytes. The FASEB
Journal 26:lb278, 2012

Chaigne-Delalande et al. Mg2+ regulates cytotoxic
functions of NK and CD8 T cells in chronic EBV
infection through NKG2D. Science 341:186-91, 2013

Bircan et al. Successful management of primary
hypomagnesaemia with high-dose oral magnesium citrate:
a case report. Acta Paediatr. 95:1697-9, 2006

Acknowledgments

Jenny Smith for the articulation and understanding that not all Magnesium deficiencies are the same.

Vanessa Hitch for taking this idea and giving incredible structure to the Types of deficiencies that occur in the community.

Cover and illustrations by Kieran Ochsenham

ABOUT THE AUTHOR'S

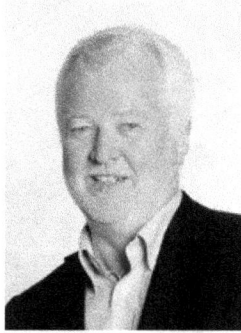

Prof. Dr. rer. nat. Jürgen Vormann

Born 1953, studied Science of Nutrition at the University Hohenheim, Stuttgart, Germany, where he also earned his Doctorate in Pharmacology and Toxicology of Nutrition.

He achieved the "Habilitation" for Biochemistry at the Institute of Molecular Biology and Biochemistry, University Clinics Benjamin Franklin, Free University Berlin, where he has the position of an extraordinary Professor. Main work areas are: biochemistry and pathophysiology of pharmacologically active food ingredients, acid-base-metabolism.

Prof. Vormann is head of the Institute for Prevention and Nutrition (IPEV) in Ismaning/Munich, Germany. Among others Prof. Vormann was president of the German Soc`iety for Magnesium-Research, Chairman of the Gordon Research Conference "Magnesium in Biochemical Processes and Medicine", Ventura, USA, and is in the advisory board of various nutrition organizations.

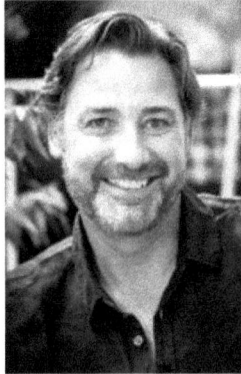

Peter Ochsenham N.D., D.B.M., Dip. Hom.

Peter's early life was dedicated to the delivery of low invasive therapy to individuals for healthcare. He is trained in all facets of Natural Healthcare, including Nutrition, Herbal Medicine, Homeopathy, Body therapy including Myofascial release, Dry Needling, as well as NLP, Hypnosis and Breathwork. However he would say his most important tool in practice was his whiteboard!

Peter's mission is to provide a platform for people to be given self-empowering options and messages for their health choices. For Peter the healthcare practitioner is the "promise" for the future of every person they see – and the message they give holds the invitation to enhance the life,"power" and embrace responsibility for greater wellbeing. Peter realizes this journey is unique to each individual and is as much about mindset, beliefs and empowerment as it is about physical activities.